HOME WORKOUT GUIDE

A COMPREHENSIVE GUIDE TO WEIGHT LOSS AND MUSCLE BUILDING

NICOLE SMITH

Table of contents

Conclusion

Introduction

Home workouts are becoming increasingly popular due to the convenience and flexibility they offer. Home workouts allow you to exercise whenever and wherever you choose, without the need for expensive equipment or a gym membership.

Home workouts are an effective way to lose weight, build muscle, and stay in shape without having to set foot in a gym, it can also be tailored to fit your individual goals and lifestyle.

Welcome to Home workouts guide! Whether you're looking to shed those extra pounds or build muscles, this book will give you the resources and tools you need to reach your fitness goals.

This book is designed to provide a comprehensive guide on how to create and execute an effective home workout routine for weight loss and muscle building. You'll learn how to design a program that fits your individual needs, and how to make it as effective as possible.

We'll discuss the benefits of home workouts, and how they can help you reach your fitness goals. We'll also cover the different types of exercises you can do, as well as how to properly perform them and how to adjust them to suit your needs and preferences. You'll learn how to create a balanced program that will challenge your body and get you the results you're looking for.

This book is designed to be a comprehensive guide for both beginners and experienced fitness enthusiasts alike. With this guide, you'll have the resources and tools you need to start your journey towards a healthier and stronger you.

Chapter 1

Understanding weight loss and muscle building

Weight loss and muscle building are two of the most common goals for many people, they are both important for overall health and fitness. Weight loss is the process of burning more calories than you consume. To achieve this, you need to create a caloric deficit. This can be done by reducing the amount of calories you consume, increasing the amount of physical activity you do, or a combination of both. When done correctly, weight loss can help you achieve healthier body weight, reduce your risk of chronic diseases, and improve your overall health and well-being.

Muscle building, on the other hand, is the process of increasing muscle mass. This is usually done through resistance training, such as lifting weights or using resistance bands. Building muscle can help you increase your strength and improve your overall physical performance. It can also help you burn more calories, even when you're at rest. To achieve both weight loss and muscle building, you need to create a balanced diet and exercise plan. Eating a balanced diet that includes all the essential nutrients and enough protein can help you lose weight and build muscle.

Weight loss and muscle building should include bodyweight exercises, strength training, and cardio exercises. Bodyweight exercises are excellent for strength and conditioning and can be used to tone and build muscle. Strength training can help build muscle and increase your strength. Cardio exercises are activities that raise your heart rate and increase your breathing rate. Cardio exercises also help to burn calories and fat, making them ideal for weight loss and maintenance.

You should also focus on getting enough sleep each night to help your body recover and rebuild muscle.

Chapter 2

The principles of workout

Understanding the principles of workouts is the key to an effective exercise program. To be successful in any kind of physical activity, you need to have a clear understanding of the fundamentals of exercise. This includes the basics of how your body moves, the types of fitness goals you can set, and what type of equipment you should use.

The first principle of a workout is understanding your body's biomechanics. This means understanding how your body moves, what muscles are involved in each movement, and how they interact with each other. This is important to know because it can help you identify which exercises will be most effective for your particular body. It can also help you determine the best way to target specific muscles and areas of the body.

The second principle of workout is setting fitness goals. This involves identifying what you want to achieve, such as getting stronger, losing weight, or improving your endurance. Once you have established your goals, you can then create a workout plan that is tailored to your specific needs. This includes choosing the right exercises, sets, and reps for each muscle group and understanding the amount of rest you need between workouts.

The third principle of workout is understanding the types of equipment you should use. Depending on what type of workout you are doing, different types of equipment will be needed. For instance, if you are focusing on strength training, then you will need different equipment than if you are doing aerobic activity. It is important to know the various types of equipment available, as well as how to use them safely and effectively.

Finally, the fourth principle of a workout is understanding the importance of rest and recovery. This involves allowing your body to rest between workouts and giving yourself time to recover from intense workouts. Proper rest and recovery are essential for building muscle and avoiding injury.

By understanding the principles of workouts, you will be able to create an effective exercise program that is tailored to your specific goals and needs. With the right knowledge and dedication, you can reach your fitness goals and lead a healthier life.

Equipment for weight loss and muscle-building workouts at home include:

1. Resistance bands: Resistance bands are great for providing resistance to your body as you perform a variety of exercises.

They can also be used for stretching and yoga.

**2.	Dumbbells	life	kettlebells:** Dumbbells and kettlebells are great for building strength and muscle. They can be used for a variety of exercises, from squats and lunges to shoulder presses and bicep curls.

3. Exercise mat: An exercise mat is essential for any home workout. It provides a comfortable surface for stretching, planks, and other floor exercises.

4. Stability ball: Stability balls are great for adding an extra challenge to your workout. They can be used for core and balance exercises as well as stretching and yoga.

5. Jump rope: Jumping rope is an effective cardio exercise that can help you burn calories and build endurance.

6. Foam roller: Foam rollers are great for relieving tight muscles and increasing blood flow. They can also be used for core and balance exercises.

7. Medicine ball: A medicine ball is a weighted ball used for a variety of strength and conditioning exercises. It is typically about the size of a basketball and is filled with sand or another dense material. Medicine balls also provide resistance to help increase strength and muscular endurance.

Chapter 3

Benefits of working out

1. Improved mental health: Exercise releases endorphins, which are a natural mood booster. Regular exercise has been linked to improved concentration and memory, as well as reduced stress and anxiety.

2. Improved physical health: Working out regularly can help to strengthen your muscles, increase your flexibility, reduce your risk of injury, improve your posture, and help you maintain a healthy weight.

3. Weight loss: One of the most notable benefits of working out is the potential to lose weight. Regular physical activity helps to burn calories, which can lead to weight loss when combined with a healthy diet. Exercise can also help to boost your metabolism, making it easier to lose weight and keep it off. Additionally, regular exercise can help to reduce body fat, which can further contribute to weight loss. With a regular workout routine, you can achieve your weight loss goals and maintain a healthy weight.

4. Muscle tone: Muscle tone is one of the many benefits of working out. It is the amount of tension in your muscles even when they are not actively being used. When you exercise, your muscles become stronger and more toned, leading to improved posture and a more toned appearance. Working out also increases the size of your muscle fibers, which helps to give your body a firmer, more toned look. Regular exercise can also help to reduce body fat, which further increases your muscle tone.

5. Improved sleep: Regular exercise helps to regulate your sleep cycle, allowing you to fall asleep and stay asleep for longer periods. Exercise can help to reduce stress levels, which can lead to better quality sleep.

Additionally, exercise raises your body temperature, and as your body cools down afterward, it can trigger sleepiness. Exercise can also help to reduce nighttime restlessness and improve overall sleep quality. So, if you're having trouble sleeping, try exercising regularly to help improve your sleep.

6. Increased energy: Regular exercise helps to make your body stronger and more efficient at using energy, allowing you to accomplish more with less fatigue. It also helps to increase circulation, allowing your body to more easily transport oxygen and nutrients to the cells that need them most. This improved circulation helps to improve your overall energy levels. Exercise also helps to reduce stress and improve sleep, both of which can leave you feeling more energized throughout the day.

7. Improved posture: Regular exercise helps to strengthen your core muscles, which helps to improve your posture. Good posture helps to relieve stress on your joints and spine, which can prevent pain and discomfort.

8. Improved self-confidence: Exercise and physical activity can help boost your self-esteem and self-confidence, as it can help you to feel better about your body, your abilities, and your overall well-being. When you exercise, your body releases endorphins, which are hormones that make you feel good and improve your mood. Exercise can also help you to look and feel better, which can give you a boost of self-confidence.

9. Improved flexibility: It can help you move more efficiently and reduce the risk of injury, especially in activities such as running and sports. Stretching before and after exercise can help your muscles become more flexible, allowing you to move with greater ease and range of motion. By increasing flexibility, you can also improve your posture and reduce the risk of strain and discomfort.

10. Improved cardiovascular health: Working out can help lower your risk of heart disease, improve your cholesterol levels, lower your blood pressure, and help you maintain a healthy weight. Regular exercise can also help improve your circulation, reduce stress, and increase your energy levels. All of these benefits can help reduce your risk of cardiovascular disease and improve your overall health.

Chapter 4

Strength training workouts

1. Push-ups: Push-up exercises are a great way to build strength and tone your muscles. It's a very simple exercise that can be done almost anywhere and requires no special equipment. The basic push-up involves lying face down on the ground and raising your body up and down by pushing your arms against the ground.

2. Squats: Squats are a great way to add strength and power to your lower body and can be done with or without weights. To do squats, stand with your feet shoulder-width apart and your toes pointing forward. Slowly bend your knees and lower your body down as if you were sitting in a chair. Make sure to keep your back straight and your core engaged. Hold the position for a few seconds before slowly returning to the starting position. Squats can be done with or without weights and can be adapted to increase difficulty.

3. Lunges: To do a lunge, stand with your feet hip-width apart, then step forward with one foot while keeping your torso upright. Lower your body until your front thigh is parallel to the floor and your back knee is just above the floor. Push up through your front heel to return to the starting position. Lunges can also be done by stepping backward, or side-to-side to target different muscles. Be sure to keep your core engaged throughout the exercise to get the most benefit.

4. Tricep dips: Tricep dips are a great exercise for strengthening and toning your upper arms. They involve using your body weight to work the triceps muscle group, located at the back of the upper arm.

The exercise is performed by sitting on the edge of a bench or chair, with your hands placed palms-down on the edge. Your arms should be straight, and your feet should be flat on the floor. Then, you lower your body down until your elbows bend at a 90-degree angle, and then push back up to the starting position. Tricep dips can be modified to increase the difficulty by adding weight or changing the angle of your body.

5. Calf raises: To do standing calf raises, stand with your feet shoulder-width apart, and raise your heels off the ground. Hold the position for a few seconds, then lower your heels back to the floor. For an added challenge, add weights to your calves.

To do seated calf raises, sit in a chair with your feet flat on the floor. Raise your heels off the floor, hold for a few seconds, then lower your heels back to the floor. Again, you can add weights to your calves for an added challenge.

6. Plank: This exercise involves holding your body in a straight line while supporting your weight on your hands and toes. Plank exercises can be done in a variety of ways, and they can be modified to fit individual abilities. To get the most benefit from plank exercise, hold the position for 30 seconds to 1 minute and repeat several times. The more reps you do, the more you will benefit.

7. Incline push-ups: This exercise is performed by placing your hands on an elevated surface such as a bench or chair, and then pushing your body off the ground. This exercise can be modified by adjusting the elevation and angle of the surface.

8. Glute bridge: The Glute Bridge is a compound exercise that is performed by lying on your back with your feet flat on the floor, knees bent, and arms out to the side. Then, you press your heels into the floor and lift your hips up and off the floor, squeezing your glutes and hamstrings as you lift. Hold for a few seconds then lower your hips back to the floor.

9. Step-ups: Step-ups are a great way to exercise your lower body. They are a full-body exercise, working your quads, glutes, and calves. Step-ups can also help improve your leg strength and endurance.

To do a step-up, stand in front of a step or platform and step up with one foot. Push through your heel as you come up and then return to start. Repeat with your other foot. You can increase the intensity of the exercise by adding weight or speed.

10. Reverse lunge: To perform the exercise, stand with feet hip-width apart and take a step back with the right foot. Lower your body by bending the left knee until it is almost touching the ground. Push through the left heel to return to the starting position and repeat on the opposite side. Make sure to keep the torso upright and the weight on the front heel during the exercise. This exercise can be modified by using dumbbells or a barbell for added resistance.

11. Wall sits: They involve sitting with your back against a wall and your feet slightly out in front of you. To do a wall sit, stand with your back against a wall and your feet slightly out in front of you. Slowly lower your body downward until your thighs are parallel to the floor. Hold this position for 30-60 seconds, then return to standing. You can add intensity to the wall sit by holding a weight in your hands.

12. Chair dips: They are a simple bodyweight exercise that can be done anywhere with a sturdy chair or bench. To perform a chair dip, stand in front of the chair and place your hands on the edge of the seat. Bend your elbows to lower your body until your elbows form a 90-degree angle. Then, press up to return to the starting position. Start with 1-3 sets of 8-12 repetitions. Be sure to keep your back close to the chair and your elbows tucked in close to your body.

13. One arm row: To perform the one arm row exercise, stand with your feet shoulder-width apart and hold a weight in one hand. Bend at the hips and lower your torso until it is nearly parallel to the floor. Keep your back straight and your core engaged throughout the exercise.

Once your torso is parallel to the floor, row the weight up to your side using your back muscles, keeping your elbow tight to your body. Lower the weight until your arm is straight and repeat for the desired number of repetitions.

14. Hyperextension: To perform a hyperextension, start by lying face down on a flat surface with your feet flat on the floor. Place your hands behind your head and then slowly raise your upper body off the ground until your spine is in a straight line. Hold the position for a few seconds and then return to the starting position. Hyperextensions should be done with caution and can be made more challenging by adding weights or resistance bands.

15. Side plank: It is an isometric exercise, meaning that the muscles remain contracted throughout the exercise.

To perform a side plank, begin by lying on your right side with your right elbow directly beneath your shoulder and your legs extended. Make sure your left foot is behind your right foot. Then, slowly raise your hips off the floor while keeping your core and glutes engaged. Hold this position for 10-30 seconds, then switch sides. Repeat this exercise three to four times on each side for best results.

16. Burpees: The burpee is performed by starting in a standing position and then quickly dropping into a squat position with your hands on the ground. From the squat position, jump your feet back into a plank position, perform one push-up, then quickly jump your feet back into the squat position. Finally, jump up into the air as high as you can before repeating the entire sequence. Burpees are a great way to get a full body workout in a short amount of time.

17. Mountain climbers: To perform this exercise, start in the plank position with your arms and legs straight. Then, bring one knee up towards your chest while keeping the other leg straight, and then switch legs. Keep alternating back and forth at a quick pace. Make sure to keep your core engaged and back flat.

18. Reverse crunch: This exercise is performed by lying flat on your back, with your knees bent and feet flat on the floor. Then, you lift your hips off the ground, bringing your knees toward your chest. You then lower your hips back down to the floor, keeping your knees close to your chest. This exercise can be modified for different fitness levels and can be used as a part of a full-body workout.

19. Jumping jacks: To do jumping jacks, start in a standing position with your feet together and your arms at your sides. As you jump, spread your legs out wide and raise your arms above your head. When you land, bring your feet back together and lower your arms. Repeat as many times as desired.

20. Russian twist: To do the Russian Twist, begin in a seated position with your feet flat on the floor and your knees bent. With your torso upright, twist your upper body to the right and then to the left. Make sure to keep your shoulders off the floor and your abs engaged throughout the entire motion. You can add weight to the exercise by holding a medicine ball or dumbbell in your hands. This will increase the intensity and challenge your core even more.

21. Bicep curls: To perform this exercise, stand with your feet shoulder-width apart and hold a weight in each hand. Keeping your elbows close to your sides, curl your arms up toward your shoulders and then lower back down. Make sure to keep your back straight and your core engaged throughout the exercise. This exercise can be done for both high reps with lighter weights or low reps with heavy weights.

22. Shoulder press: To perform the shoulder press, hold a barbell with your hands slightly wider than shoulder-width apart. Then press the bar up, straightening your elbows and fully extending your arms overhead. Lower the bar back down, keeping your arms just slightly bent. Repeat for desired reps.

23. Abdominal crunches: To perform a crunch, start by lying on your back with your feet flat on the floor and your knees bent. Place your hands behind your head and tuck your chin into your chest. Tighten your abdominal muscles and lift your shoulders off the floor, keeping your lower back on the ground. Exhale as you lift and inhale as you lower. Lower your shoulders back down to the starting position and repeat.

24. Bent-over row: To perform a bent-over row, stand with your feet hip-width apart, hinge your hips back, and lower your chest parallel to the floor while keeping your back straight. From here, grab the weight with both hands and row it up to your chest while squeezing your shoulder blades together. Make sure to keep your core engaged and maintain a neutral spine throughout the entire movement. Squeeze your shoulder blades at the top of the movement, and slowly lower the weight back to the starting position. This exercise is great for building strength, improving posture, and developing a stronger back.

25. Medicine ball slams: The basic technique of medicine ball slams is to hold a medicine ball with both hands and raise it above your head. Then throw it down onto the ground as hard as you can. The impact of the ball will cause your entire body to move and engage the core, arms, shoulders, and legs. Repeat the same process 10-15 times and you will see great results.

26. V-ups: The exercise can be performed by lying flat on your back and then lifting your legs and arms off the floor. Simultaneously, crunch your upper and lower body together to form a "V" shape. Hold this position for a few seconds before returning your arms and legs to the starting position. This exercise can be modified to make it easier or more challenging. It's also a great way to mix up your ab routine!

27. Woodchops: To perform a woodchop, stand with your feet shoulder-width apart and hold a medicine ball, dumbbell, or a weight plate in both hands. Twist your torso to one side, and as you twist, bend your knees slightly and raise the weight up and across your body. Keep your arms straight and your core engaged as you do this. Then reverse the motion, twisting your torso in the opposite direction and bringing the weight back to the starting position. You can perform the woodchop in a variety of directions, including side-to-side, up and down, and front-to-back.

28. Crossover crunches: To perform this exercise, start by lying on your back with your knees bent and your feet planted firmly on the floor. Place your hands behind your head and lift your shoulders off the ground, while simultaneously crossing your right leg over your left leg. Bring your left elbow to meet your right knee and then lower back down. Repeat the same motion, but on the opposite side, bringing your right elbow to meet your left knee. Try to do 10-15 repetitions on each side for best results.

29. Shoulder Tap: This exercise helps build stability in your shoulders and upper body, and can be performed as part of a full-body workout. To do shoulder taps, stand up straight and lift one arm and tap the opposite shoulder with your hand. Make sure to keep your core engaged and your back straight. Repeat with the other arm and continue alternating between the two arms. You can also do this exercise while in a plank position, which will require more balance and stability. Shoulder taps can be done with weights or without, depending on your fitness level.

30. Bent Over Row: This exercise involves bending over at the hips, keeping the back straight, and pulling a weight towards your midsection. To perform this exercise correctly, you need to keep your back in a neutral position and maintain a slight bend in your knees. Make sure to keep your arms close to your body as you pull the weight up. This exercise can be done with a barbell, dumbbell, or resistance band.

Chapter 5

Body weight workouts

1. Plank: Plank exercise is a great way to strengthen your core and increase overall body strength. It involves holding your body in a plank position, which is a static position where you support your body weight on your hands and toes. This position works your core muscles, arms, shoulders, and back, and can help improve posture, balance, and coordination. Plank exercises can be done as part of a regular workout routine or as a stand-alone exercise. To get the most benefit from plank exercise, hold the position for 30 seconds to 1 minute and repeat several times. The more reps you do, the more you will benefit.

2. Burpees: The exercise begins with a plank position, and then you drop into a squat position. From the squat position, you jump up and reach your hands up to the ceiling. Finally, you drop back into the plank position and repeat the sequence. Burpees are great for burning calories and helping to build strength and endurance.

3. Single-Leg Deadlift: To perform a single-leg deadlift, stand on one foot with your other leg slightly bent and in front of you. Slowly hinge forward at the hip and lower your torso until it is parallel to the floor. Engage your core and keep your back straight as you lift your torso back up to the starting position. Make sure to keep your weight on your heel and your knee slightly bent throughout the movement. You can also add a kettlebell or dumbbell to increase the intensity of the exercise.

4. Tricep Dips: To perform a tricep dip, start by sitting on the edge of a bench or chair with your hands on the edge of the seat. Lift your body off the seat, with your arms straight, and lower your body until your upper arms are parallel with the ground. Hold for a few seconds, then push back up to starting position. This can be repeated for 8-12 repetitions.

5. Calf Raises: To perform calf raises, start by standing upright with your feet hip-width apart and then slowly raise your heels off the ground as high as you can while keeping your legs straight. Hold this position for a few seconds before slowly lowering your heels back down. You can also perform calf raises while holding onto a barbell or dumbbell for added resistance.

6. Bicycle Crunches: To perform a bicycle crunch, start by lying on your back with your knees bent and feet flat on the ground. Place your hands behind your head, keeping your elbows wide. Then, crunch up, bringing your right elbow to your left knee while extending your right leg straight out. Switch sides, bringing your left elbow to your right knee while extending the left leg. Continue alternating sides for the desired number of repetitions.

7. Superman: It involves lying face down on the floor with your arms and legs extended. Then, you lift your upper body and legs off the floor while keeping your arms and legs straight.

8. Plank jacks: To perform a plank jack, begin in a plank position with your elbows on the ground and your feet shoulder-width apart. Keeping your back straight, jump your feet out to the sides and then quickly back to the starting position. Repeat this movement for the desired number of repetitions.

9. Mountain Climbers: To do the exercise, start in a plank position, with your hands and feet on the ground. Then, alternate bringing one knee up towards your chest, and then back to the starting position. Repeat this motion on the other side, and keep alternating sides for the desired number of repetitions.

10. Reverse Lunge: To perform reverse lunges, stand with your feet hip-width apart and take a big step back with one leg. Bend both knees to lower your body until your back knee is just above the ground. Push off your back leg to return to the starting position and repeat with the opposite leg. Reverse lunges can be done with or without weights. Start with body weight and progress to adding dumbbells or a barbell to challenge yourself.

11. Spiderman Pushup: To perform the Spiderman Push-Up, begin in a high plank position with your hands below your shoulders. Bend your elbows to lower your chest towards the ground. As you lower your chest, bring your right knee forward and up towards your right elbow. Pause here for a second before pressing back up to the starting position. Repeat the same motion with your left leg and left elbow. Continue this alternating motion for the desired number of reps.

12. Jumping Jacks: To perform jumping jacks, start with your feet together and your arms at your sides.

Then, jump up into the air, and as you do, spread your legs out to shoulder width and your arms out to shoulder height. Make sure to keep your back straight. As you land, bring your feet back together and your arms back down to your sides. Repeat for the desired amount of time or number of reps. Jumping jacks are a great way to get your heart rate up and get your body ready for any activity.

13. High Knees: To perform this exercise, stand with your feet hip-width apart and lift one knee towards your chest while keeping the other foot on the ground. Switch legs and repeat. Increase the intensity by running in place while lifting your knees higher. This exercise can be done anywhere and is a great way to get your heart rate up and burn calories.

14. Skater Hops: To perform skater hops, start by standing with your feet slightly wider than hip-width apart. Bend your knees and reach down with your arms straight. Begin hopping from one foot to the other, alternating feet and keeping your body low. Make sure to keep your back straight and your arms extended. Try to reach as far as you can with each hop. Do this exercise for 30 seconds and then rest for 30 seconds. Repeat this sequence 3-5 times.

15. Squat Jumps: They are a plyometric exercise that helps to build strength and power in the lower body. To perform a squat jump, start by standing with feet shoulder-width apart and then bending your knees and lowering your hips until your thighs are parallel to the ground. Then, explosively jump as high as you can, extending your arms up and out over your head. Land softly, absorbing the impact with your legs as you bend your knees and return to the starting position. Make sure to warm up and stretch before performing any plyometric exercises to avoid injury.

16. Pushup Jacks: To perform a push-up jack, start in a plank position with hands slightly wider than shoulder-width apart. Lower your body until your chest is just above the ground. As you push yourself back up, jump your feet out to the sides and clap your hands together above your head. Jump your feet back to the start and lower your body into the next push-up.

17. Toe Tap: To do this exercise, stand with your feet hip-width apart and your arms at your side. Lift your right leg and tap your toes to the ground in front of you. Then switch legs and do the same on the other side. Do this for 30 seconds and repeat. This exercise can be modified by adding light dumbbells or resistance bands for an extra challenge.

18. Frog Jumps: To do a frog jump exercise, start from a standing position with your feet shoulder-width apart and your arms at your sides. Lower yourself into a squat position, and then jump up as high as you can while extending your arms out to the sides. Land softly and then repeat the jump.

19. Reverse Crunch: To perform this exercise, lie flat on the floor or on an exercise mat, with your hands either behind your head or resting on your chest. Lift your legs off the floor, bringing your knees towards your chest. Keep your lower back pressed into the floor and your abs contracted as you slowly lower your legs back to the floor. Repeat this motion for the desired number of repetitions.

20. Split Squat: To perform a split squat, stand with one foot forward and the other foot back. Lower your body until the back knee almost touches the ground, then drive up through the heel of your front foot to return to the starting position. You can also hold dumbbells or a barbell for added intensity.

21. Reverse Plank: This exercise is performed by lying on your back and lifting your hips off the floor while balancing on your hands and feet. Your arms should be straight and your feet should be slightly wider than shoulder-width apart. You should hold this position for 30-60 seconds, then lower your hips and repeat.

22. Spiderman Climb: To do the exercise, you begin in a push-up position with your hands and feet on the floor. Then, you will move one hand up and outward, and the other hand down and inward, creating a Spiderman-like motion. You will then repeat this motion with the opposite hands, alternating sides each time.

23. Single Leg Squat: To perform the exercise, stand on one foot and slowly lower your body by bending the knee of your supporting leg. Make sure to keep your back straight and your chest up. Once you have reached a comfortable depth, push back up to the starting position. Repeat the exercise for the desired number of repetitions before switching to the opposite side.

24. Glute Kickback: To do a glute kickback exercise, start by getting into a kneeling position on the floor. Place your hands on the ground and keep your back flat. Engage your core muscles, and then kick one leg straight out behind you, keeping your heel in line with your knee. Pause when your leg is parallel to the ground, and then slowly return to the starting position. Repeat the same movement with your other leg.

Be sure to keep your core engaged throughout the entire movement, and your back straight. You can also increase or decrease the intensity of the exercise by adjusting the range of motion, speed of movement, or number of repetitions.

25. Fire Hydrant: Start by standing with your feet hip-width apart and the dumbbells in each hand. Bend your knees slightly and hinge forward at the hips until your upper body is parallel to the ground. Shift your weight to one leg and lift the other leg off the ground. Keep your core engaged and your back straight.

From this position, perform a lateral abduction movement with the lifted leg, as if you were pushing a fire hydrant out to the side. You can do this with or without the dumbbells. When you are finished with one side, switch legs and repeat.

26. Reverse Shoulder Tap: To perform this exercise, start by standing with your feet shoulder-width apart and your hands at your sides. Then, reach one hand behind your back and tap the opposite shoulder with the back of your hand. After completing the tap, return your hand to the starting position. Repeat this motion with the opposite arm.

This exercise can be made easier by reducing the range of motion and increasing the number of repetitions. It can be made more challenging by increasing the range of motion and decreasing the number of repetitions.

27. Single Leg Glute Bridge Pulse: This exercise requires you to lie on your back with one leg bent and your foot flat on the floor. The other leg should be extended and lifted off the floor. From this position, you will raise your hips off the floor and pulse your hips up and down. To increase the intensity of the exercise, you can add weight to your hips, hold the bridge for longer periods, or increase the number of pulses.

28. Wide Pushup: It is performed by placing your hands wider than shoulder-width apart on the floor and then pushing your body up and down. This exercise can also be modified to target different muscles by adjusting the width of the arms.

29. Donkey Kicks: This exercise is simple yet effective and can be done by anyone. To do the exercise, start on all fours with your hands directly under your shoulders and your knees under your hips. Then, lift one leg up and back so that it is parallel to the ground and your knee is bent at 90 degrees. Hold the position for a moment before slowly returning to the starting position. Repeat with the other leg. You can challenge yourself by adding hand weights or ankle weights for extra resistance.

30. Single Leg Hop: To perform the single leg hip exercise, stand on one leg and brace your core. Slowly lower your body down until your thigh is parallel to the ground. Hold for a few seconds, then slowly return to the starting position. Make sure to keep your back straight and your core tight throughout the exercise.

This exercise can be performed with or without weight, depending on your fitness level. Make sure to keep your knee soft and avoid locking it. This exercise can be performed for multiple reps, or as a single, long hold.

31. Squat Hold: To perform the exercise, slowly lower yourself into a squat position and hold the position for as long as you can. Make sure you keep your chest and back upright and your abdominals engaged. The longer you can hold the squat, the better.

When performing a squat hold, the feet should be placed shoulder-width apart and the chest should be kept upright. The arms should be held out in front or at the sides. The back should remain straight and the abdominals engaged. The weight should be centered in the heels and the toes should be pointed slightly outward.

32. Inchworm: To perform the inchworm exercise, start in a standing position with your feet shoulder-width apart. Bend over and place your hands on the floor in front of you, then walk your hands out as far as you can until your body forms a straight line from your hands to your feet. Hold this position for a few seconds, then walk your hands back towards your feet and stand up.

33. Heel Touches: It is a simple exercise that can be done virtually anywhere and requires minimal equipment. To do the heel touches exercise, start by lying on your back with your feet flat on the floor and your knees bent. Place your arms at your sides with your palms facing down. Then, slowly lift your right leg off the floor and touch your right heel to your left hand. Return your right leg to the starting position, and then switch sides, touching your left heel to your right hand. Repeat this motion for the desired number of repetitions.

34. Lateral Shuffle: To do the lateral shuffle, start by standing with feet shoulder-width apart. Step laterally to the right with the right foot, keeping the left foot in place. Then, step to the left with the left foot, overlapping the right foot. Repeat the lateral steps in this fashion, staying low and keeping the chest up. Focus on keeping the good form as you move laterally. This exercise can be performed at a moderate or fast pace, depending on your fitness level.

35. Bird dog: To perform the Bird Dog exercise, start in a tabletop position with your hands and knees on the floor. Keeping your back flat and abs tight, extend your right arm and left leg straight out, and hold for a couple of seconds. Return to the starting position and repeat on the opposite side. Continue alternating between the right and left sides for the desired number of repetitions.

Chapter 6

Cardio workouts

1. Jumping jacks: Jumping jacks are a classic exercise that can be done anywhere and are great for getting your heart rate up. They are a full-body, dynamic exercise that works your arms, legs, core, and even your cardiovascular system.

To do jumping jacks, start with your feet together and your arms at your sides. Then, jump out with your feet wider than shoulder-width apart and your arms up in the air. Jump back to the starting position and repeat for the desired number of repetitions. Make sure to keep your core tight and your back straight throughout the exercise.

2. Squat jumps: To do a Squat Jump, start by standing with your feet shoulder-width apart and your hands on your hips. Then, lower into a squat position with your arms reaching out in front of you. Make sure your back is straight, your chest is up, and your knees are aligned over your toes.

From here, jump as high as you can, reaching your arms up in the air. As you land, lower back into the squat position. Make sure to land softly to reduce the risk of injury. Do 10-15 repetitions for 3-4 sets for best results.

3. Burpees: They involve a combination of strength and cardio, working your entire body. They are a great way to burn calories, build muscle and improve your cardiovascular endurance.

To do a burpee, start in a standing position, then squat down and jump back into a push-up position. Do one push-up, then jump your feet back to your hands and jump into the air. Repeat this sequence for as many repetitions as you **can.**

4. Mountain climbers: It is also a great way to burn fat, build endurance, and increase your cardiovascular health.

To perform mountain climbers, start in a pushup position with your arms fully extended and your feet shoulder-width apart. Then, alternate pushing one knee towards your chest, while keeping the other leg straight. Continue to alternate legs for 30 seconds. To make the exercise more challenging, try to increase the speed and intensity of the exercise.

5. Running: Running is a great form of exercise for both physical and mental health. It helps to improve your cardiovascular fitness, strengthens your muscles, and can help to boost your mood. It also helps to reduce stress and can provide an opportunity for social interaction.

When running, it is important to warm up and stretch before starting, as this helps to reduce the risk of injury. It is also important to wear comfortable and supportive shoes and to stay hydrated throughout your run.

6. Heel touch: To perform the heel touch exercise, begin in a seated position with your feet flat on the floor. Place your hands behind your head, elbows wide, and lift your chest off the floor. Lift your right leg and bring your heel up towards your left hand. Reach around the back of your head with your left hand and touch your right heel. Hold for a few seconds and then switch sides. Repeat for 10 to 15 repetitions.

7. Speed walking: Speed walking is a great low-impact exercise that can be done almost anywhere, and it's easy to fit into your daily routine. To get the most out of your speed walking workout, make sure you have the proper form and speed. Start with a slow pace and gradually work up to a faster pace as your fitness level increases. Make sure to keep your arms bent at the elbow and your hands relaxed, and try to keep your shoulders relaxed.

8. Running the stairs: When running the stairs, you should always use proper form and be sure to warm up first. Start by walking up the stairs slowly, then gradually increase your speed as you go. Focus on pushing off with each step and using your arms to help propel you up the stairs. Whenever possible, switch up the direction you are going in to work your calves and glutes in different ways.

Remember to cool down after your stair running session and make sure to stretch your muscles. This will help to prevent any injuries and help you recover faster.

9. Swimming: Swimming is a great way to exercise your body and get in shape. It is a low-impact activity that puts minimal stress on your joints and can help to improve your overall strength, flexibility, and endurance. Swimming is also a great way to burn calories and can help with weight loss.

10. Cycling: Cycling is a low-impact exercise that can be done almost anywhere, and it's suitable for people of all ages and fitness levels. Cycling is a great form of aerobic exercise, which can help to improve your overall cardiovascular health, strengthen your muscles and bones, and increase your energy levels.

11. High knees: To do high knees, stand with your feet hip-width apart. Lift your right knee to your chest, keeping your knee bent. Immediately switch legs and lift your left knee to your chest. Continue alternating legs, keeping a steady rhythm, and maintaining an upright posture. Aim to lift your knees as high as you can each time.

12. Skipping: It is a great way to increase your cardiovascular fitness, improve your coordination and agility and tone your muscles. Skipping is also a great way to burn calories and lose weight.

For the best results, it is important to use the right technique. Start by standing with your feet shoulder-width apart and hold the rope in each hand. Swing the rope up and over your head and jump over it when it comes around. Make sure your arms move in time with your feet as you jump.

13. Step-ups: To do a step-up, stand in front of a box or step, and place one foot on the box. Step up onto the box, using your heel to push off the ground, and bring your other foot up to meet it. Step back down with the same foot, and repeat on the other side. Start with bodyweight step-ups and add weight once you've mastered the movement.

14. Power walking: Power walking is a type of exercise that combines walking with an aerobic workout. It is a great way to get your heart rate up and burn calories while strengthening your muscles. Power walking involves taking longer strides than regular walking and pumping your arms to add intensity to the workout. It is a form of aerobic exercise that can help you lose weight and improve your overall fitness.

15. Kettlebell swings: These involve swinging a kettlebell from side to side and then up and down while maintaining a strong core and upright posture.

16. Box jumps: They involve jumping onto a box or other raised platform, then quickly jumping off and landing on the ground. Box jumps work the entire body, including the core, glutes, quadriceps, hamstrings, and calves.

17. jogging: Jogging is a great aerobic exercise that can help improve your overall health. It can help you lose weight, increase your cardiovascular fitness, and strengthen your muscles and bones. Jogging is low impact, so it can be done safely by most people.

It's easy to do, and all you need to get started is a good pair of running shoes and comfortable clothes. When jogging, it's important to start slowly and gradually increase your intensity and distance as your fitness level improves.

18. Split jumps: To do a split jump, start standing with your feet together. Jump up and split your legs so that one foot is forward and one is back. When you land, absorb the impact and immediately jump up again, switching your legs so the other foot is forward. Do this for 30 seconds to one minute, depending on your fitness level.

19. Leg raises: When performing leg raises, the basic technique involves lying on your back with your legs straight and slightly apart. You then lift your legs off the ground until they are at a 90-degree angle and then lower them back down. If you are using weights, you can hold them in your hands while performing the exercise.

20. Bear crawls: To do a bear crawl, start in a position that looks similar to a push-up. Your hands should be directly below your shoulders, and your feet should be directly below your hips. From here, move your right hand and left foot forward at the same time, followed by your left hand and right foot. Continue this pattern for about 10 repetitions or for a set length of time.

21. Sumo squat to toe: To do the exercise, start by standing with feet wider than hip-width apart and toes pointing out. Squat down as low as you can while keeping your chest up, back straight, and weight in your heels. As you stand up, lift your left leg and reach your toes out in front of you. Repeat on the other side to complete one rep. Keep your chest up and core engaged throughout the exercise for maximum benefit.

22. Straight-leg bicycles: To do this exercise, sit on the edge of a chair or bench and extend your legs, so they are straight out in front. Lift one leg off the floor, keeping the other leg straight, and begin pedaling the air with your extended leg. Move your leg in a circular motion, and pedal for 10 to 15 repetitions. Switch legs and repeat. This exercise can be done with light weights for added resistance.

23. Forward jump: This exercise is typically performed by standing with feet shoulder-width apart and then jumping forward as far as possible. It is important to remember to land softly and absorb the shock of the landing to prevent any injuries.

It is also beneficial to perform this exercise in a variety of angles and directions to target different muscles and increase the overall effectiveness of the exercise.

24. Dance exercise: Dance exercise can also be a great way to get your heart pumping and burn calories. It can be done alone or in a group setting and can be tailored to any fitness level. Whether you're looking for a fun way to get fit or just a way to move your body, dance exercise can be a great option.

25. Speed skater: To perform the exercise, you should stand with your feet together and your arms extended out in front of you. Then, jump laterally to the right, landing on your right foot while bringing your left leg behind you and crossing your arms. Push off your right leg to return to the starting position, and then repeat the move on the left side. It is important to keep your movements fluid and controlled and make sure to keep your core engaged throughout the exercise.

26. Step back jacks: To do Step Back Jacks, start in a standing position with your feet together. Jump up and land with your feet apart. Simultaneously, as you jump up, bring your arms up above your head and as you land, bring your arms back down to your sides. Jump up again, this time landing with your feet together. Repeat this move for a full minute.

27. Butt kicks: To do butt kicks, start in a standing position. Then, raise one knee towards your chest, and kick your heel towards your butt. Repeat with the other leg. Do 15-20 repetitions on each side. As you do the exercise, keep your back straight and your abs tight.

28. Tuck jump: To perform a tuck jump, start from a standing position and then jump up, bringing your knees up to your chest, and tucking your feet up towards your glutes. When airborne, fully extend your legs back out and land softly on both feet, making sure to keep your chest up and your core tight throughout the entire movement. Tuck jumps can be a challenging exercise, so it is important to start with a low number of repetitions and gradually increase as your strength progresses.

29. plank jacks with shoulder taps: To perform this exercise, start in a plank position with your arms fully extended and your feet together. Next, jump your feet out to the side, like a jumping jack, and tap your opposite shoulder with the opposite hand. Then, jump your feet back together and repeat the movement, this time tapping the other shoulder with the other hand. Continue to alternate sides for the desired number of repetitions.

30. Star jump: This exercise requires you to stand with your feet hip-width apart and your arms at your sides. To begin the exercise, you will jump up and spread your legs out to either side while simultaneously raising your arms above your head. As you land, return your legs and arms to the starting position. Keep repeating the exercise for a minute or two.

Star jumps are great for improving overall fitness, as they challenge the major muscle groups of the body. They can also be a great way to get your heart rate up to burn calories and fat.

Chapter 7

Safety tips for home workout

1. Warm up and cool down: Before and after every workout make sure to do a proper warm-up and cool down. This will help to properly prepare your body for the upcoming workout and help to prevent any potential injuries.

2. Use proper form: Proper form is key when it comes to any exercise. Make sure to focus on the quality of your movements and use proper form throughout the entire exercise. This will help to ensure that you get the most out of your workout and stay safe.

3. Listen to your body: Make sure to listen to your body and stop if you are feeling any pain or discomfort. If you experience any sharp or sudden pain, stop immediately and consult your doctor.

4. Have an open space: Make sure to have an open space for your workout, free from any obstacles or hazards. Clear the area of anything that may get in the way of your workout and could potentially cause an injury.

5. Wear proper athletic shoes: Wear proper athletic shoes when doing any type of exercise. Having the right shoes can help to reduce the chance of injuries and provide more stability while working out.

6. Don't overexert yourself: Don't overexert yourself while working out. Pushing yourself too hard can lead to fatigue and injuries. Make sure to take breaks if needed and don't push yourself past your limits.

7. Hydrate: Make sure to stay hydrated while working out. Dehydration can cause fatigue, dizziness, and other health problems.

8. Use the right equipment: Make sure to use the right equipment for your workout. Using the wrong equipment can lead to injuries and can make the workout more difficult.

9. Have a spotter: If you are doing any exercises that involve lifting weights or any other type of heavy lifting, make sure to have a spotter. This will help to ensure safety and will reduce the chance of any potential injuries.

10. Stretch: Make sure to stretch before and after every workout. This will help to reduce any stiffness and help to prevent any potential injuries.

11. Wear comfortable clothes: Wear comfortable clothes that won't restrict your movements or cause any discomfort.

12. Know your limits: Make sure to know your limits and don't push yourself too hard. If you are a beginner, start slow and gradually increase the intensity of your workouts.

Conclusion

Home Workout Guide is a comprehensive guide to help you reach your goals for weight loss and muscle building. With the right approach and dedication, you can make the most of your body and achieve the healthy physique you desire. No matter your starting point, this guide will help you progress and reach the level of fitness you desire. With the right attitude and commitment, you can achieve your goals and achieve the body you've always wanted.